COLOSTOMY DIET COOKBOOK

I0429922

Delicious And Nutrient-Packed Friendly Recipes For Savoring Life After Surgery, Wellness And Healthy Lifestyle

DR LUCAS KAYCE

DISCLAIMER

This book about illness and nutrition is not meant to replace expert medical advice, diagnosis, or treatment; rather, it is meant purely for informational reasons. This book's content is founded on broad concepts and recommendations for managing diseases and nutrition.

Before adopting any major dietary or lifestyle changes, readers are recommended to speak with a qualified healthcare provider, such as a licensed physician or registered dietitian, especially if they have pre-existing medical concerns. Everybody has different health demands, so what works for one person might not work for another.

The use of the information provided in this book may have unfavorable repercussions or consequences, for which the author and publisher disclaim all liability. No disease is meant to be identified, treated, cured, or prevented by the information provided.

The book may include contain references to medical literature or research findings; however readers are urged to independently confirm this material and contact reliable sources.

It is important to remember that the fields of nutrition and medicine are always changing, and that new findings could have an impact on the advice offered in this book. As a result, readers are urged to keep up with the most recent advancements in healthcare and, when in doubt, seek professional counsel.

By reading this book, readers agree that they are in charge of their own health decisions and release the author and publisher from any liability arising from the use of the material in the book, whether direct or indirect.

TABLE OF CONTENTS

COLOSTOMY DIET OVERVIEW 11

   CONCERNING COLOSTOMY...11

   THE VALUE OF A DIETARY SPECIALIZATION 12

CHAPTER ONE 14

   COMPREHENDING COLOSTOMY 14

   WHAT IS A COLOSTOMY?...14

   MANY COLOSTOMIES TYPES 14

   HAVING A COLONOSCOPY...15

CHAPTER TWO 18

   CONSUMPTION OF FOOD AND COLOSTOMY.....................18

   NUTRITION'S SIGNIFICANCE 18

   DIETARY NEEDS FOR PATIENTS WITH COLOSTOMIES 19

   TYPICAL PROBLEMS AND THEIR FIXES..............................20

CHAPTER THREE 22

   CREATING A COLOSTOMY DIET THAT IS HEALTHY 22

   AN INTRODUCTION TO A COLOSTOMY-FRIENDLY DIET 22

   MEAL PREPARATION AND PORTION MANAGEMENT.........23

CHAPTER FOUR 26

   INGREDIENTS THAT ARE COLOSTOMY-FRIENDLY 26

   FRUITS AND VEGETABLES...26

   SOURCES OF PROTEIN 27

   GRAINS AND CARBS..27

   DAIRY AND SUBSTITUTES 28

   FATS AND OILS 29

CHAPTER FIVE..30

   COOKING METHODS FOR MEALS THAT ARE COLOSTOMY-FRIENDLY....30

      HOW TO COOK FOOD TO MAKE IT DIGESTIBLE.................................30

      DELICIOUS SEASONINGS THAT DON'T HURT..................................31

      RECIPE ADAPTATIONS FOR PATIENTS WITH COLOSTOMIES..............32

CHAPTER SIX..34

   EXAMPLE MENUS...34

      IDEAS FOR BREAKFAST...34

      LUNCH IDEAS...35

      OPTIONS FOR DINNER..36

      RECIPES FOR SNACKS..37

      CELEBRATE SPECIAL EVENTS AND MINGLE AT PARTIES AND GET-TOGETHERS..38

      ADVICE FOR DINING OUT..39

      RECIPES THAT ARE COLOSTOMY-FRIENDLY FOR EVENTS...................40

CHAPTER SEVEN...42

   COLOSTOMY AND HYDRATION..42

      HYDRATION...42

      DRINKS APPROPRIATE FOR PEOPLE WITH COLOSTOMIES.................43

      HELP FOR MAINTAINING PROPER HYDRATION..........................45

CHAPTER EIGHT...48

   HANDLING INTESTINAL PROBLEMS.....................................48

      HANDLING GAS...48

      HANDLING CONSTIPATION..48

      REDUCING ODOR...49

CHAPTER NINE 52

  ASPECTS OF EMOTION AND PSYCHOLOGY 52

    HANDLING NUTRITIONAL SHIFTS 52

    DEVELOPING A POSITIVE RELATIONSHIP WITH FOOD 53

    LOOKING FOR ASSISTANCE 55

ABOUT THE BOOK

The "Colostomy Diet Cookbook" is an indispensable tool for those managing their colostomy; it provides thorough guidance for constructing a healthy, well-balanced diet that is specific to their requirements. The opening portions clarify the numerous varieties of colostomy and the daily struggles faced by those who have this illness, offering crucial insights into the notion. The importance of implementing a customized diet is emphasized, stressing its function in fostering general health and digestive well-being.

The book covers the basic knowledge of colostomy, including its physical and psychological components. The book highlights the critical role that nutrition plays in the lives of those with colostomies, making comprehension of the nutritional requirements even more important. It goes beyond just listing difficulties; rather, it provides workable answers to typical food problems, guaranteeing a comprehensive strategy for handling dietary worries.

The book helps readers create a balanced colostomy diet, is the core of the book. Along with the essentials, it offers a thorough examination of important nutrients, portion management, and efficient meal planning. Beyond theory, it lists elements that are suitable for colostomies, providing a wide variety of choices in fruits, vegetables, cereals, proteins, and other foods.

The book's advice on appropriate cooking methods and sample meal plans to help with the daily application of a colostomy-friendly diet put practicality front and center in the following chapters. Understanding that social settings and special events can pose particular difficulties, it provide advice on how to handle get-togethers and stress the significance of staying properly hydrated.

In addition to the medical issues, the book discuss the psychological and emotional effects of having a colostomy. It promotes a healthy connection with food and offers coping mechanisms in recognition of the effects on mental health.

The "Colostomy Diet Cookbook" is more than just a standard recipe book, to put it simply. It serves as a thorough manual that provides information, encouragement, and useful guidance to enable people with colostomies to not only meet their dietary demands but also lead happy, full lives.

COLOSTOMY DIET OVERVIEW

CONCERNING COLOSTOMY

In the field of medicine, some illnesses call for special treatments and lifestyle modifications to protect the health of the afflicted parties. A surgical treatment known as a colostomy, which creates a stoma by redirecting a part of the colon through a hole in the abdominal wall, is one example of such an intervention. The rerouting of fecal matter to a collecting bag linked to the stoma is usually necessary when a portion of the colon is sick or injured. The length of a colostomy depends on the underlying medical problem and the general health of the patient.

Numerous conditions are treated with colostomies, such as congenital anomalies, severe injuries, inflammatory bowel illnesses (including Crohn's disease or ulcerative colitis), and colorectal cancer. The development of a colostomy has a significant impact on a person's day-to-day functioning since it modifies the regular course of bowel motions.

Along with physical adjustments, living with a colostomy also requires emotional and psychological adjustments. To adjust to the new circumstances around their digestive health, patients frequently need assistance and instruction.

THE VALUE OF A DIETARY SPECIALIZATION

A specific diet is crucial for preserving the health and comfort of those who have a stoma, especially when combined with the surgical component of colostomy. Bypassing the colon modifies the digestion process, which impacts how well water and nutrients are absorbed.

Because of this, medical practitioners frequently advise dietary changes to meet the unique requirements of those who have colostomies. For people with colostomies, understanding and following a unique diet is essential to avoiding difficulties, guaranteeing adequate nutrition, and improving their overall quality of life.

Patients with colostomies usually follow a specific diet plan that takes into account things like fiber consumption, staying hydrated, and avoiding items that can cause blockages in the stoma or increased gas output. Dietitians, medical professionals, and patients themselves must collaborate and receive instruction to strike a balance between a variety of healthy foods and potential health risks. Although adjusting to life with a colostomy is not easy, people can have happy, healthy lives after surgery if they receive the correct information and assistance.

We go into the complexities of both colostomy and the importance of a specific diet in this discussion, illuminating the medical, psychological, and nutritional facets that support the comprehensive care of those who have had this surgical operation.

CHAPTER ONE

COMPREHENDING COLOSTOMY

WHAT IS A COLOSTOMY?

A colostomy is a surgical technique in which a section of the large intestine (colon) is directed to the skin's surface through the creation of an incision in the abdominal wall. Waste can pass through this incision, called a stoma and a colostomy bag is fitted to collect and handle the evacuated stool. Rerouting the natural flow of feces is often required for colostomies due to diseases, injuries, or congenital disorders that affect the bottom section of the digestive system.

MANY COLOSTOMIES TYPES

There are various colostomy kinds and the type that is best for you will depend on where the stoma is located and how much of the colon is affected. Ascending colostomies, transverse colostomies, and descending or sigmoid colostomies are three frequent classifications based on the area of the colon from which the stoma is formed. A transverse colostomy is made from the transverse colon, a descending or sigmoid colostomy is formed from the descending or sigmoid colon, and an ascending colostomy is constructed by bringing the end of the ascending colon to the stoma. A person's medical condition and the amount of necessary operations determine the type of colostomy they will have.

HAVING A COLONOSCOPY

Living with a colostomy necessitates adjusting to new routines and ways of controlling body processes. A colostomy can have a profound emotional and psychological impact on a person since it can cause emotions of humiliation, self-consciousness, or anxiety in social situations. To assist people in adjusting to their new situation and developing confidence in their ability to manage their colostomy, appropriate education, and support from medical professionals are essential.

To manage a colostomy and avoid consequences like skin irritation and infection, routine maintenance of the stoma and surrounding skin is necessary. For comfort and convenience of usage, selecting the right colostomy equipment is crucial, especially the kind of colostomy bag. Colostomy bags can be drainable or closed-end, and they are available in a variety of forms, including one-piece and two-piece systems. The choice is based on the individual's unique demands and personal preferences.

Dietary changes could also be required to control the consistency of the feces and lessen the chance of gas or odor. Healthcare providers, including nurses and dietitians, are essential in offering advice on food selection, caring for stomas, and resolving any issues that may come up during the transition phase.

For those who are living with a colostomy, support groups, and counseling programs are invaluable tools because they provide a forum for exchanging stories, asking for guidance, and establishing connections with people who are aware of the difficulties related to this drastically different treatment. Having a strong support system made up of friends, family, and medical experts can greatly improve the general well-being and quality of life of people who have colostomies. To support people in managing not just the physical but also the emotional and social elements of living with a colostomy, education, emotional support, and practical aid are crucial.

CHAPTER TWO

CONSUMPTION OF FOOD AND COLOSTOMY

NUTRITION'S SIGNIFICANCE

Maintaining general health and well-being is heavily dependent on nutrition, which is particularly important for those who have a colostomy. Following colostomy surgery, the body's ability to digest and absorb vital nutrients is changed, therefore it's critical for patients to closely monitor what they eat. Sufficient nutrition improves the patient's quality of life, aids in preventing problems, and promotes the body's healing process.

Maintaining energy levels, encouraging tissue healing, and strengthening the immune system all depend on proper nutrition. Patients with colostomies may experience particular difficulties with digestion and nutrient absorption, so it's critical to create a diet that is well-balanced and tailored to their requirements. A meal high in nutrients not only speeds up the healing process but also helps shield against deficits brought on by stomach system alterations.

DIETARY NEEDS FOR PATIENTS WITH COLOSTOMIES

Changes in bowel function are common in colostomy patients, and these changes might impact the digestion and absorption of nutrients. To make sure they fulfill their nutritional needs, they must concentrate on a few dietary factors. It is generally advised to consume a diet high in fiber to control bowel motions and avoid constipation. To prevent possible problems like blockages, some colostomy patients may need to restrict their intake of specific types of fiber.

Consuming protein is essential for maintaining muscle mass and repairing tissue, particularly during the recuperation stage. Patients with colostomies should include lean protein sources in their diet, such as fish, poultry, eggs, and plant-based proteins. Maintaining proper hydration is equally important since it promotes healthy digestion, reduces the risk of stoma-related issues, and helps prevent dehydration.

For general health, vitamins and minerals are necessary, and individuals with colostomies should monitor their consumption of important nutrients such as vitamin B12, calcium, and iron. Supplementation may be advised in some situations to address particular deficits that can develop as a result of altered digestive function.

TYPICAL PROBLEMS AND THEIR FIXES

Patients with colostomies may experience a range of nutritional difficulties, such as controlling fluid intake, addressing possible weight fluctuations, and worrying about specific meals making them uncomfortable. A typical difficulty is getting used to a new diet that takes into account the altered digestive tract. Foods that can irritate or produce gas around the stoma should be recognized and, if required, avoided.

Keeping the right amount of hydration is another difficulty. Since certain colostomy patients may be more susceptible to dehydration than others, it's important to keep an eye on fluid intake and modify it as necessary. Maintaining adequate hydration prevents problems such as electrolyte imbalances and enhances general health.

Another factor to take into account is weight control, since certain individuals may have changes in their weight as a result of impaired nutrient absorption. Any variations in weight can be addressed with routine weight monitoring and dietary modifications made under the supervision of a healthcare provider or nutritionist.

Colostomy patients require a comprehensive approach to feeding. This entails being aware of and adjusting to the changed digestive system, maintaining a diet that is nutrient-dense and well-balanced, and addressing particular issues with tailored remedies.

CHAPTER THREE

AN INTRODUCTION TO A COLOSTOMY-FRIENDLY DIET

To ensure that people with colostomies can keep adequate nutrition while maintaining their digestive health, it is important to carefully examine several elements while creating a balanced diet for them. The foundation of a diet suitable for people with colostomies is selecting foods that are simple to digest, unlikely to clog pipes and enhance general health.

Focusing on a well-balanced diet that consists of a range of nutrient-rich foods is one important component. This can assist in supplying the body with the nutrients it needs and promote general wellness. A variety of fruits, vegetables, lean proteins, nutritious grains, dairy products, or dairy substitutes should be included in the diet of those with colostomies. It can be helpful to choose high-fiber foods, such as whole grains and specific fruits and vegetables, but it's important to introduce them gradually to gauge tolerance.

Essential Elements for Patients with Colostomies

Essential nutrients are essential for maintaining the health of those who have colostomies. To avoid dehydration and preserve regular bowel movements, it is essential to drink enough water. Drinking enough water can also promote overall digestive health and help avoid obstructions. Patients with colostomies need to be mindful of the vitamins and minerals they consume, such as calcium, iron, and vitamin B12. These nutrients are essential for preserving bone health, and energy levels, and the avoidance of shortages that may compromise general health.

MEAL PREPARATION AND PORTION MANAGEMENT

Meal planning and portion control are crucial elements of a diet that is colostomy-friendly. Throughout the day, eating smaller, more frequent meals can aid with discomfort management and digestion. Controlling portion sizes is crucial to prevent overtaxing the digestive system, since larger meals may heighten the likelihood of experiencing gas, bloating, or discomfort. Planning meals includes selecting foods that are easily tolerated and introducing new ingredients one at a time to rule out any potential allergies or triggers.

Colostomy patients must be extremely aware of their body's signals and steer clear of foods that could aggravate their condition. Maintaining a food journal can help you monitor your eating habits and spot trends in your digestion, bowel movements, and general health.

Furthermore, seeking advice from a medical expert or a certified dietician with ostomy care experience can offer tailored recommendations and assistance based on specific needs and preferences.

Choosing nutrient-rich foods, concentrating on important nutrients, exercising portion control, and meal planning are all important components of creating a nutritious diet for people with colostomies. Colostomy patients can maintain a nutritious and well-balanced diet that promotes their general health and well-being by paying attention to their unique tolerances and preferences.

CHAPTER FOUR

INGREDIENTS THAT ARE COLOSTOMY-FRIENDLY

FRUITS AND VEGETABLES

Including a range of fruits and vegetables in a diet that is suitable for a colostomy is crucial to preserving general health and well-being. These foods contribute to a balanced nutritional profile and support digestive health by providing essential vitamins, minerals, and fiber. Choosing easier-to-digest fruits and vegetables can be advantageous for people who have a colostomy. Steamed or cooked vegetables like apples, zucchini, and carrots may be easier on the stomach. Fruits with seeds and peels, such as melons and bananas, are also frequently well-tolerated.

To ensure a colostomy-friendly diet that supports optimum digestion, it's important to experiment with different cooking techniques and prepare fruits and vegetables in ways that reduce potential irritation.

SOURCES OF PROTEIN

Because protein is essential for tissue regeneration and general bodily function, it should be a part of any diet designed with a colostomy. To reduce discomfort and potential difficulties, people with colostomies may choose to prioritize easily digestible protein sources while making their selections. Fish, poultry, and tofu are examples of lean proteins that might be wise choices. Instead of frying, it's best to prepare proteins by grilling, baking, or steaming because these techniques are usually easier on the digestive tract. Eggs cooked to perfection and creamy nut butter are other healthy ways to increase your protein intake without overtaxing your digestive system.

GRAINS AND CARBS

When selecting grains and carbs that are suitable for a colostomy, it is important to give priority to those that are quickly digested and high in fiber and vital nutrients. For people who have a colostomy, white rice, cooked pasta, and refined grains like white bread may be better since they are less likely to irritate or clog the ostium. Soluble fiber foods, including oatmeal and cooked peeled potatoes, can be added to promote regularity of the stool without sacrificing comfort.

Individual tolerance levels can vary, so it's important to watch portion amounts and how the body reacts to various grains and carbohydrates.

DAIRY AND SUBSTITUTES

You can include dairy products in your diet if you have a colostomy, but you should be aware of any potential post-surgery lactose intolerances or sensitivities. Choosing low- or lactose-containing options, including dairy-free yogurt or lactose-free milk, can help colostomy patients avoid experiencing gastrointestinal distress. To keep your bones healthy, you can also include non-dairy calcium sources like leafy greens, tofu, and fortified plant-based milk in your diet instead of just traditional dairy products.

It's great to try a variety of dairy and nondairy choices to see what suits each person's digestive system the best.

FATS AND OILS

A colostomy-friendly diet should contain healthy fats for energy and overall nutritional balance. Selecting fats that are simple to break down, such as those in nuts, avocados, and olive oil, can supply necessary fatty acids without overtaxing the digestive system. Fried and fatty foods can be more difficult to digest and might cause discomfort, thus people who have colostomies may want to restrict their consumption of these items. Cooking techniques like baking, grilling, or sautéing with little to no oil can assist people who have colostomies reap the benefits of healthy fats without jeopardizing their digestive health. Maintaining digestive comfort requires watching portion sizes and paying attention to how the body reacts to various fat sources.

CHAPTER FIVE

COOKING METHODS FOR MEALS THAT ARE COLOSTOMY-FRIENDLY

HOW TO COOK FOOD TO MAKE IT DIGESTIBLE

When cooking for people who have a colostomy, it's important to concentrate on techniques that maximize digestibility and reduce discomfort. It is advised to use gentle cooking methods like steaming, boiling, and baking since these aid in the breakdown of food without placing undue strain on the digestive tract.

These techniques guarantee that the final meals are tender, simple to chew, and easy on the stomach, improving the comfort of digestion and nutrient absorption for colostomy patients.

Including steaming in the cooking process has special advantages. This technique maintains the delicate texture of the ingredients while preserving their inherent flavors and minerals. For people who have a colostomy, steamed veggies, fish, and poultry are great options because they are easy to digest while maintaining their nutritional value. Boiled foods can have a softer consistency that facilitates digestion, such as pasta, cereals, and some vegetables.

DELICIOUS SEASONINGS THAT DON'T HURT

Meal preparation for colostomies doesn't have to sacrifice flavor. But to prevent irritability, seasonings must be used carefully. Choose seasonings and herbs that enhance flavor without upsetting the stomach. Herbs such as rosemary, thyme, basil, and oregano can improve the flavor of a variety of foods without being unduly harsh on the stomach. Furthermore, sparingly utilizing fresh herbs like ginger and garlic can add a taste boost without irritating the skin.

Dishes that are extremely spicy or highly seasoned should be avoided by colostomy patients as they may cause digestive problems. Taste can be preserved while expanding palate diversity by experimenting with moderate, well-tolerated spices. For a cool variation, it's also a good idea to add citrus components like lemon or lime, which can add brightness to food without irritating the palate.

RECIPE ADAPTATIONS FOR PATIENTS WITH COLOSTOMIES

Making deliberate changes to ingredients and preparation techniques is necessary when modifying recipes to meet the demands of colostomy patients. For instance, it can be simpler to digest vegetables if they are peeled or cooked to a softer consistency. Selecting fish, poultry, and other lean proteins over fatty meats reduces the chance of experiencing stomach pain.

Refined grains can be substituted for whole grains in recipes to lower the amount of fiber, as too much fiber might be difficult for colostomy patients to digest. Reducing the number of large meals to three smaller ones throughout the day can also help with better digestion and absorption of nutrients.

Additionally, for those who have lactose intolerance—a typical problem for those who have a colostomy—

incorporating lactose-free or low-lactose options can be useful. To create recipes that are tailored to each patient's unique dietary requirements and tastes and to ensure that they have a satisfying and well-balanced gastronomic experience, healthcare specialists and nutritionists must be consulted.

CHAPTER SIX

EXAMPLE MENUS

IDEAS FOR BREAKFAST

A balanced breakfast is crucial to provide the body with nutrients and energy for the day. To provide you with energy throughout the morning, try including a variety of macronutrients, such as proteins, carbs, and healthy fats. Good options include a Greek yogurt parfait with fruits and granola or a protein-rich omelet with veggies. Nuts and berries on top of oatmeal or whole-grain cereals add fiber, which promotes healthy digestion and a feeling of fullness.

Smoothies with mixed fruits, leafy greens, and a protein source like yogurt or protein powder can be a healthy and portable option for people on the go. Another simple yet filling choice is avocado toast on whole-grain bread, which provides complex carbohydrates and healthy fats. Make sure your breakfast has the right combination of nutrients to power your body for the day by customizing it to your dietary requirements and taste preferences.

LUNCH IDEAS

Midday is a good time to refresh and restock on nutrients with lunch. A well-balanced lunch should include a variety of lean proteins, nutritious grains, and vibrant veggies. A nutrient-dense choice is grilled chicken or tofu salads with mixed veggies and a vinaigrette dressing. A wonderful and convenient option is whole grain wraps stuffed with lean protein, fresh veggies, and avocado or hummus.

As an alternative, think about packing leftovers from dinner the night before for lunch. This guarantees a balanced meal while also lowering food waste. Lunch alternatives that are both varied and delicious include a stir-fry with a range of veggies and a lean protein source, or a quinoa bowl with roasted vegetables, beans, and a savory sauce. Keep in mind to drink plenty of water, and for extra nutrition, have a small portion of nuts or a side of fruits.

OPTIONS FOR DINNER

Dinner is a time to relax and fuel your body with a filling and healthy dish. Choose a range of protein sources, including lean meats, grilled fish, and plant-based foods like lentils or chickpeas. Combine them with healthful grains such as sweet potatoes, quinoa, or brown rice to supply complex carbohydrates for long-lasting energy.

Your dinner plate should be dominated by vegetables, which provide a variety of vitamins and minerals. Vegetables that have been roasted, steamed, or stir-fried and enhanced with herbs and spices provide your food taste and nutrition. Try experimenting with different cooking styles to keep evenings interesting. Try Asian stir-fries with colorful veggies and tofu, or grill fish and vegetables with a Mediterranean flair.

Adding a source of good fats to your dinner—like avocado or olive oil—can help with overall satiety and aid in the absorption of fat-soluble vitamins. Always remember to eat mindfully, enjoying every bite and being aware of your body's signals of hunger and fullness.

RECIPES FOR SNACKS

A healthy diet should include snacks since they provide you energy in between meals and help you avoid overindulging at meals. To stay full, pick snacks that are high in protein, good fats, and carbohydrates. Easy yet nutrient-dense options include Greek yogurt with a sprinkle of honey or a handful of nuts with a piece of fruit.

Try sliced veggies with guacamole or whole-grain crackers with hummus for a savory variation. A tiny portion of cheese with whole-grain crackers or nut butter on whole-grain toast can offer a filling combination of nutrients and flavors. Nut butter, dried fruit, and oats combine to create energy balls that are lightweight and easy to carry along.

To prevent consuming too many calories from snacks, pay attention to portion sizes. Observe your body's hunger signals and select foods that meet your dietary requirements. To encourage healthy choices when hunger strikes in between meals, think about making snack-sized servings ahead of time and keeping them easily accessible.

CELEBRATE SPECIAL EVENTS AND MINGLE AT PARTIES AND GET-TOGETHERS

Special occasions and social gatherings may be thrilling as well as difficult, particularly when it comes to navigating parties and gatherings. Knowing the social forces at work is essential. Maintaining personal boundaries while remaining friendly should be balanced. Start by introducing yourself, genuinely interested in other people, and paying attention to the atmosphere in the room.

Social interactions heavily rely on body language. Keeping your body language friendly and approachable can encourage others to start conversations. In a similar vein, recognizing cues from other people facilitates determining the right degree of interaction.

Effective party navigation requires establishing shared interests, pastimes, or life experiences with other guests.

ADVICE FOR DINING OUT

Dining out is a popular social activity, so it's important to approach it mindful of your dietary requirements as well as your tastes. Consider the group's tastes when selecting a restaurant, and make sure there are selections to suit a range of palates.

It's important to express to the waiter or chef any special dietary requirements or preferences you may have.

Portion control is yet another important consideration when dining out. To sample a range of flavors without going overboard, think about splitting plates with several people.

Eating carefully and appreciating every meal also improves digestion in addition to improving the dining experience.

RECIPES THAT ARE COLOSTOMY-FRIENDLY FOR EVENTS

Food is a major part of celebrations, and for those who have a colostomy, it's critical to discover recipes that are not only delicious but also suitable for their device. It's important to choose foods that are easy to digest and kind to the digestive tract. Well-cooked vegetables and dishes with lean proteins, like grilled chicken or fish, can be excellent options.

It's important for people who have colostomies to think about how different meals affect their ability to digest. Eating less fiber, spicy food, and elements that cause gas can all help you have a more comfortable meal. Including cooked grains, soft fruits, and easily digested proteins in meals can help strike a balance between digestion health, and enjoyment on special occasions.

In conclusion, navigating parties and gatherings successfully requires knowledge of social dynamics and the skill to strike a balance between being gregarious and respectful of others' personal space. Good communication and awareness of one's dietary requirements are important components of a satisfying dining experience. When colostomy-friendly recipes are used to celebrate significant occasions, it guarantees that those who have them can partake in the festivities without jeopardizing their digestive health.

CHAPTER SEVEN

COLOSTOMY AND HYDRATION

HYDRATION

The relevance of hydration is increased for those who have a colostomy because it is an essential component of preserving general health and well-being. Several physiological processes, such as digestion, circulation, and temperature regulation, depend critically on adequate hydration. Sustaining enough hydration is even more crucial for colostomy patients since it helps ward off problems and guarantees the best possible functioning of the digestive system.

For people who have a colostomy, staying hydrated is essential to avoid dehydration, which can result in several health problems. Electrolyte abnormalities brought on by dehydration may impair the body's capacity to effectively absorb nutrients. Patients with colostomies frequently struggle with fluid loss, and dehydration can make matters worse. This can result in consequences like kidney difficulties, constipation, and UTIs.

Furthermore, preserving the suppleness of the surrounding skin and the stoma depends on enough hydration. Dehydrated skin is more prone to irritation and can become fragile, which raises the possibility of colostomy pouch issues. Drinking enough water keeps the skin around the stoma strong and healthy, which improves the quality of life for those who have colostomies.

DRINKS APPROPRIATE FOR PEOPLE WITH COLOSTOMIES

Colostomy sufferers must choose their drinks carefully to stay hydrated without endangering the health of their digestive tract. The most obvious and widely advised source of hydration is water. It is necessary to keep the colostomy from becoming dehydrated and to make sure that the feces pass through easily. Colostomy patients should attempt to consume enough water each day to fulfill their specific needs, and they should do so consistently throughout the day.

Apart from water, additional appropriate liquids for those with colostomies are herbal teas, clear juices, and electrolyte-rich beverages. Clear liquids, like apple or cranberry juice, can supply certain vital nutrients and extra water.

Herbal teas, such as those flavored with peppermint or chamomile, are calming and generally easy on the stomach. Electrolyte-rich beverages, which might include oral rehydration solutions with specific formulations, can assist in replacing electrolytes lost through fluid loss, especially in warmer climates or after physical activity.

When choosing beverages, colostomy patients should be aware of their unique tolerances and preferences. Carbonated or caffeinated drinks might irritate some people, so it's best to cut back on your consumption if they make you uncomfortable or aggravate gas problems.

HELP FOR MAINTAINING PROPER HYDRATION

It takes deliberate effort and commitment to healthy habits to stay well hydrated, especially for those who have a colostomy. Establishing a regular drinking schedule and distributing your fluid intake equally throughout the day is one useful tactic. This strategy guarantees a steady flow of fluids to promote healthy digestion and helps avoid dehydration.

Urine color monitoring is a straightforward way to determine one's level of hydration. While strong yellow or amber hues may signify the need for higher fluid intake, pastel yellow normally indicates appropriate hydration. Patients with colostomies should strive for equilibrium and refrain from consuming too much fluids, since this may result in dehydration.

Including foods high in water content, like fruits and vegetables, in the diet can help increase the amount of fluid consumed overall. It's also a good idea to limit your consumption of diuretics like alcohol and coffee because they can cause you to lose more fluid.

For colostomy patients to obtain individualized guidance on hydration that takes into account their unique medical conditions and demands, regular communication with healthcare providers are vital. People who have a colostomy can minimize the risk of issues related to low fluid intake and increase general well-being by adopting healthy behaviors and being attentive to staying hydrated.

CHAPTER EIGHT

HANDLING GAS

A common digestive problem, gas can be uncomfortable and awkward in social situations. Finding the root causes of gas is crucial to managing it successfully. Eating some foods that cause gas, such as cabbage, beans, and carbonated drinks, can cause gas production to rise. One way to deal with gas is to include probiotics in the diet. These can help with digestion and support a balanced population of gut bacteria. Furthermore, eating mindfully and abstaining from overindulging can help reduce the buildup of gas in the digestive tract. To rule out underlying digestive issues, seeking medical advice may be important for individuals who experience persistent or severe gas.

HANDLING CONSTIPATION

The common digestive ailment known as constipation is typified by irregular bowel motions and trouble passing feces. Dietary and lifestyle choices are very important in treating constipation. It's important to be well hydrated because it facilitates regular bowel movements and softens poo. Consuming a diet high in fiber-rich foods, like fruits, vegetables, and whole grains, can help the stool pass more easily by giving it more volume. By encouraging bowel regularity, regular physical activity also supports a healthy digestive tract. If you are experiencing chronic constipation, see a doctor for a thorough assessment and individualized treatment plan.

REDUCING ODOR

Managing digestive problems entails taking care of any social issues as well as physical suffering, such as reducing the odor of bowel movements. Unpleasant scents can come from some foods, such as vegetables (like broccoli and cauliflower) that contain sulfur. Odor can be lessened by adhering to good hygiene habits, such as frequent hand washing and air freshener use. Eating foods high in chlorophyll, such as parsley or mint, can also help to balance or lessen the smell of the digestive tract. Those with severe or chronic odor problems should speak with a medical expert to determine any possible underlying causes and to obtain personalized guidance on how to take care of this area of digestive health.

To address specific issues and advance general well-being, an integrated approach to digestive health combines dietary changes, lifestyle adjustments, and, when required, expert assistance.

CHAPTER NINE

ASPECTS OF EMOTION AND PSYCHOLOGY

HANDLING NUTRITIONAL SHIFTS

Making dietary adjustments can be a complex process with both mental and physical components. When making dietary changes, people frequently experience a range of feelings, from joy and optimism to worry and annoyance. Maintaining a fine balance between addressing potential emotional issues and accepting the need for transformation is necessary to cope with these changes. It is imperative to approach dietary modifications with an attitude of self-compassion, understanding that adjustment takes time. Resilient coping strategies include controlling expectations and realizing that obstacles are a normal part of the process.

Personal preferences, cultural factors, and long-standing habits all have a role in the emotional reaction to dietary changes.

Emotional barriers can arise from a sense of deprivation or from a fear of losing out on favored foods. Taking the initiative to try new foods, play around with flavors, and look for healthier substitutes for dishes can all help reduce the emotional burden. Additionally, consulting a nutritionist or joining a support group can offer insightful advice and useful strategies for handling the psychological effects of dietary changes. Essentially, adjusting to new nutritional routines and developing emotional resilience to overcome obstacles are both necessary components of coping with dietary changes.

DEVELOPING A POSITIVE RELATIONSHIP WITH FOOD

Developing a positive relationship with food goes beyond its nutritional value and is a comprehensive process. It includes the aspects of eating that are social, psychological, and cultural. Recognizing and combating unfavorable eating-related beliefs and attitudes is necessary to cultivate a positive attitude toward food.

This could entail destroying guilt connected to particular foods, breaking through restrictive beliefs, and encouraging mindfulness during meals. Gaining awareness of one's own hunger and satiety cues is essential to fostering a healthy relationship with food because it helps people listen to their bodies and eat in a balanced manner.

Encouraging a healthy eating environment is also very important. This entails designing environments that promote mindful eating, honor the senses associated with food, and cultivate an attitude devoid of judgment regarding one's food preferences. Eating meals together with those you love can enhance the social and emotional aspects of eating and strengthen good food associations. A more sustainable and pleasurable relationship with food can be achieved by embracing variety and flexibility in diet choices, eschewing strict guidelines, and promoting a sense of empowerment in making decisions that are in line with personal preferences and wellbeing.

LOOKING FOR ASSISTANCE

Seeking support from multiple sources is often necessary when embarking on emotional and psychological journeys related to dietary changes and developing a positive relationship with food. Assistance can take many different forms, such as expert advice from dietitians, nutritionists, or mental health specialists with expertise in eating disorders. These professionals can offer individualized plans, coping techniques, and resources to help people deal with the psychological complexities of dietary changes. Additionally, asking friends and family for help can build a network of understanding and support, creating a setting where people feel appreciated for their efforts.

Getting involved in online communities or support groups centered around health and wellness can also foster a sense of belonging and common experiences. Through the chance to share struggles, celebrate successes, and exchange insights, these platforms foster a positive ecosystem that rewards constructive behavior.

It's also critical to acknowledge the emotional components of the journey and engage in self-compassion practices. Acknowledging that asking for help is strength rather than a weakness enables people to overcome obstacles and achieve long-term improvement in their emotional and psychological connections to food and dietary modifications.